SMOOTHIES FOR PANCREATIC CANCER

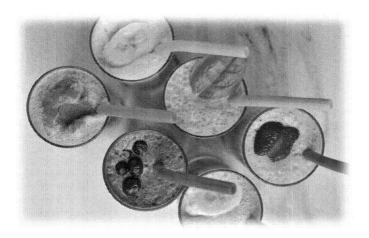

Simple Delicious Smoothie Recipes to Support and Manage Your Pancreatic Health

By

Dr. Clara Ramsey

Contents

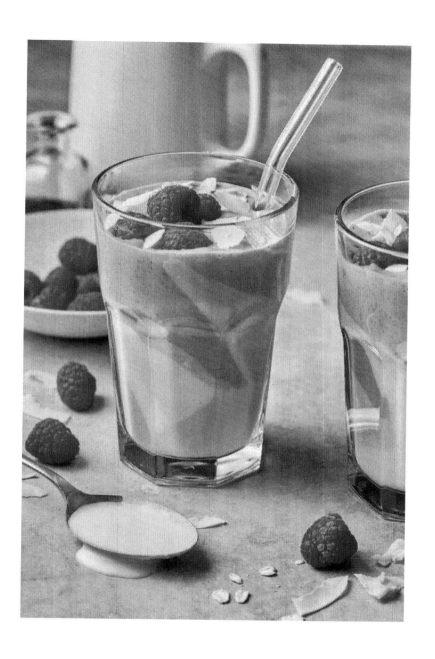

Introduction

A Simple, Delicious Way to Support Your Health

Imagine this: You're in your kitchen, and the sunlight filters through the window as you gather fresh ingredients—vibrant berries, a handful of spinach, maybe some creamy avocado or a sprinkle of chia seeds. You toss them into a blender, press the button, and in seconds, you've created something powerful; a smoothie that's not just delicious but filled with nutrients your body truly needs.

For anyone facing the challenges of pancreatic cancer, food can often feel like both a friend and an enemy. Some days, even the thought of eating seems overwhelming, and maintaining weight or energy feels like an uphill battle. But that's where smoothies come in.

This book is not just about smoothies. It's about finding a way to nourish your body with something easy to make, gentle on the stomach, and packed with the goodness that supports healing. These smoothies are designed to fuel your body with key nutrients that help you fight fatigue, promote digestion, and maintain your strength—all while being incredibly easy to digest.

Why smoothies, you want to ask?

Let me tell you a quick story. A few years ago, I had a close friend diagnosed with pancreatic cancer. Every day was a struggle—appetite issues, energy dips, and the constant worry of how to keep her body strong enough for the battle ahead. The turning point came when she discovered smoothies.

They became a lifeline, offering a soothing, nutritious, and enjoyable way to get the vitamins, minerals, and calories she desperately needed. With just a few simple ingredients, she found herself not only feeling more energized but also in control of her nutrition.

And the best part? She could customize her smoothies to suit her mood, taste preferences, and dietary needs on any given day.

So, you can be rest assure that this book is born from that experience, with a heartfelt mission: to offer you a tool that's easy to use and gives you control over what goes into your body during this challenging time.

Whether you're managing treatment side effects or just looking for a way to boost your energy and feel good, the smoothies in this book are here to support you.

Anyway, let's get blending. Each recipe in this book has been thoughtfully crafted to ensure that you're not just filling a glass—you're fueling your body with what it needs most. Plus, these smoothies are quick, simple, and (best of all) delicious. So let's make nutrition the easiest part of your day.

Let me tell you something important: when you're dealing with pancreatic cancer, every little thing you do for your body matters. Every bite, every sip, and every choice you make can either help fuel your strength or leave you feeling depleted. That's why nutrition plays such a crucial role in your health journey.

But here the thing you don't realize, food can feel complicated when your body isn't acting like it used to.

You might be asking,

"What should I eat? What should I avoid? Why do I feel so different?"

These are questions that come up all the time, and you're not alone in feeling overwhelmed by them.

I will like to share a story about a patient named Sarah.

Sarah had always been a food lover—her days revolved around colorful, hearty meals, and she found joy in cooking for her family. But when she was diagnosed with pancreatic cancer, everything changed. She lost her appetite, started to lose weight rapidly, and the foods she once loved no longer sat well with her. Food, which once brought joy, now became a source of anxiety.

After speaking with her dietitian, Sarah learned that pancreatic cancer affects how the body processes food. The pancreas plays a critical role in digesting food and regulating blood sugar, so when it's not functioning well, it's no wonder things start to feel off. Digestive issues, weight loss, and fatigue are common symptoms that many people, like Sarah, experience.

So, what's the solution?

It's a nutrition that works with your body, not against it, but before then let me tell you the power of smart nutrition.

Part One

The Power of Smart Nutrition

The right nutrition plan can help you regain control, even when so much feels out of your hands. While there's no magic food that can cure cancer, what you put into your body can make a real difference in how you feel day-to-day.

Think of it like this: your body is already working hard to fight, and the food you eat is the fuel that helps power that fight.

When we think about nutrition for pancreatic cancer, there are a few key things to keep in mind:

Gentle on Digestion: Since the pancreas helps digest food, it's important to choose foods that are easy to digest and absorb. This is where smoothies shine. With everything blended together, your body can quickly take in the nutrients without having to work too hard.

Energy Boosting: You'll want to focus on nutrient-dense ingredients that pack a lot of goodness into a small serving. When you're dealing with a reduced appetite, every sip counts. Think ingredients like leafy greens, berries, protein sources like Greek yogurt, and healthy fats like avocado.

Balancing Blood Sugar: The pancreas also helps regulate blood sugar, so keeping it steady is important. Low-glycemic fruits, healthy fats, and proteins help keep energy levels stable, avoiding the sugar crashes that can leave you feeling even more tired.

Anti-inflammatory: Inflammation is common in cancer patients, and certain foods can actually help reduce inflammation in the body. Ingredients like turmeric, ginger, and leafy greens are anti-inflammatory superheroes you can easily add to your smoothies.

A Professional's Take on Cancer and Nutrition

I once spoke with a dietitian who worked exclusively with cancer patients, and she told me something that really stuck. She said, "It's not just about getting calories into the body; it's about getting the right kind of calories." That means prioritizing foods that give your body the vitamins, minerals, proteins, and fats it needs to stay strong during treatment.

She recalled working with a patient named Mark, who was undergoing chemotherapy for pancreatic cancer. Mark had lost significant weight, and his energy was at an all-time low. His body was craving nutrients, but eating solid food made him feel sick. That's when they turned to smoothies.

Together, they crafted smoothies that were easy to sip and full of nutrient-rich ingredients—things like spinach for iron, flaxseed for omega-3s, and bananas for potassium. Slowly, Mark began to feel more energized. The smoothies weren't just a meal replacement—they were a lifeline, helping him keep his strength up during treatment.

Why Smoothies Work So Well

When you think about it, smoothies are kind of like the Swiss Army knife of nutrition. They're versatile, quick to make, and, best of all, you can pack them with all sorts of powerful ingredients without sacrificing taste.

And when you're dealing with pancreatic cancer, they can be a lifesaver, especially on days when you don't feel like sitting down for a big meal.

But here's the trick: not all smoothies are created equal. The key is to choose ingredients that give you the most bang for your buck, nutritionally speaking.

In this book, you'll find recipes that are specially designed to be easy on the stomach, energizing, and full of the nutrients that your body craves during treatment.

Just like Sarah, Mark, and many others, you too can take control of your nutrition. It doesn't have to be complicated, and it doesn't have to feel like a burden. With a bit of guidance and the right ingredients, you can create smoothies that not only taste great but also help you feel stronger, more energized, and ready to face the challenges ahead.

As you turn the pages of this book, think of it as a tool to help you care for yourself. Each recipe is carefully crafted to support your body's unique needs during pancreatic cancer treatment. We'll cover everything from energizing breakfast smoothies to calming blends for those tough days when your appetite just isn't there.

Together, we'll make nutrition something you look forward to again. After all, your body deserves to be fueled with love, care, and the best ingredients we can find. Now, let's blend up something amazing!

The Role of Smoothies in Healing and Recovery

A Simple Yet Powerful Approach

Let's face it: when you're dealing with pancreatic cancer, food can feel like a challenge. Some days, just thinking about a full meal can feel exhausting. Other days, your appetite is nowhere to be found, and getting the right nutrients into your body seems like an uphill battle. But there's a secret weapon in your kitchen that can help you nourish and support your body without the overwhelm: smoothies.

Smoothies are more than just a convenient option—they're a powerful tool in your healing and recovery journey. Think of them as liquid nutrition that's gentle on your system, easy to prepare, and packed with exactly what your body needs to fight, heal, and recover. But don't just take my word for it—let me share a story about a patient who discovered the magic of smoothies during her cancer treatment.

A Story of Healing

I once worked with a patient named Linda, a strong woman in her early 60s who had been diagnosed with pancreatic cancer. Like many others, the treatments took a toll on her body. She felt constantly fatigued, had difficulty digesting food, and was rapidly losing weight. One of her biggest struggles was maintaining enough energy to get through the day, and traditional meals just weren't cutting it.

She enter smoothies. After talking to her dietitian, Linda started incorporating smoothies into her daily routine, and it was a game-changer. Each smoothie was carefully designed to provide her body with essential nutrients—protein for strength, healthy fats for energy, and fiber for digestion.

Slowly, Linda began to feel a shift. Not only were the smoothies easy to consume, but they also gave her a steady stream of energy without making her feel overwhelmed by large portions of food.

What Linda found most comforting was the variety and flexibility that smoothies offered. On days when she felt nauseous, she could sip on a light, hydrating smoothie made with cucumber, watermelon, and ginger. On days when her energy was low, she could boost her intake with a more substantial smoothie packed with protein powder, spinach, and avocado. And the best part? These smoothies didn't just fill her stomach—they gave her a sense of control over her nutrition during a time when everything else felt uncertain.

How Smoothies Support Healing and Recovery

I can tell you that smoothies are the unsung heroes of pancreatic cancer recovery for a number of reasons.

Here's why they work so well:

Easy on Digestion: With pancreatic cancer, digestion can be tricky. Since the pancreas plays a key role in breaking down food, many patients struggle with discomfort, bloating, or indigestion after meals.

Smoothies, however, are pre-blended and easy to digest. By blending fruits, vegetables, proteins, and healthy fats, you're essentially giving your body a head start on the digestion process. This makes smoothies a much gentler option compared to heavy or solid meals.

Customizable Nutrition: Every day with cancer is different—your energy levels, appetite, and digestive comfort can change at the drop of a hat. Smoothies allow you to adjust your nutrition based on how you're feeling. Whether you need more protein, fiber, or hydration, you can tweak your smoothie ingredients to meet your needs in that moment. And if there's a flavor or texture you love (or can't stand), smoothies can be easily adjusted to suit your preferences.

Nutrient-dense in Every Sip: When appetite is low, it's critical to pack as much nutrition into each bite—or in this case, each sip—as possible. Smoothies give you the chance to combine multiple nutrient-rich ingredients into one drink. From leafy greens to nuts and seeds, you're getting a variety of vitamins, minerals, and antioxidants in every serving. It's like having a multivitamin that actually tastes good!

Energy and Hydration Boost: One of the hardest challenges during pancreatic cancer treatment is fatigue. Because smoothies can be loaded with energy-boosting ingredients like protein, healthy fats, and fruits, they can help you maintain more consistent energy levels throughout the day.

Plus, by adding liquids like coconut water or almond milk, you're staying hydrated, which is especially important for digestion and overall health.

Key Nutrients for Pancreatic Health

What to Include in Your Smoothies

Now that we've covered why smoothies are such a great option, let's dive into the specific nutrients that support pancreatic health. By focusing on these key ingredients, you can create smoothies that not only taste great but also provide the essential building blocks for recovery.

Protein: Protein is vital for repairing tissues and maintaining muscle mass, which is especially important if you're losing weight or feeling weak during treatment. Great protein sources for smoothies include Greek yogurt, protein powder, nut butters, and even tofu. Adding protein can help you feel fuller and provide the energy you need to stay strong.

Healthy Fats: Healthy fats are crucial for energy and maintaining weight during cancer treatment. Avocados, flaxseed, chia seeds, and nut butters are fantastic options to blend into your smoothie. These fats are also anti-inflammatory, which can help reduce inflammation in the body and support healing.

Fiber: Maintaining good digestive health can be challenging with pancreatic cancer, but fiber can help keep things moving smoothly. Ingredients like spinach, berries, chia seeds, and oats are excellent sources of fiber, aiding digestion and supporting a healthy gut.

Antioxidants: Pancreatic cancer and its treatments can cause oxidative stress in the body, but antioxidants help fight off free radicals and promote healing. Berries (like blueberries and strawberries), leafy greens (such as kale and spinach), and even spices like turmeric are packed with antioxidants that can boost your immune system and support recovery.

Vitamins and Minerals: Nutrient-rich ingredients like leafy greens, bananas, and nuts provide essential vitamins and minerals that your body needs to function at its best.

For example, spinach is a great source of iron and magnesium, while bananas are rich in potassium, which helps balance electrolytes and support muscle function.

Hydration: Staying hydrated is essential for every aspect of your health, especially during cancer treatment. Adding ingredients like coconut water, cucumber, or watermelon to your smoothies helps keep you hydrated, supporting your kidneys, digestion, and overall well-being.

Ready to Blend?

Smoothies are more than just a meal—they're a way to reclaim your nutrition and make eating feel manageable again. With each sip, you're giving your body the nutrients it needs to heal, recover, and thrive. So whether you're craving something light and refreshing or rich and filling, you can count on smoothies to deliver exactly what you need.

Now, let's get blending! These recipes are designed to fuel your body, soothe your system, and make the journey just a little bit easier. Together, we're going to blend our way to better health.

Part Two

Tips for Making the Perfect Smoothie

Blending Your Way to Delicious Nutrition

Making the perfect smoothie is part science, part art—and 100% about what you enjoy. The beauty of smoothies is that they're incredibly versatile, which means you can play around with flavors, textures, and ingredients until you find your go-to blend.

Whether you're trying to pack in as many nutrients as possible or create something that satisfies your sweet tooth, making a great smoothie is easier than you might think.

Let's dive into a few simple tips that will help you master the art of smoothie-making, while keeping things fun and delicious!

1. Start with a Solid Base

The foundation of a great smoothie starts with a liquid base. It's what keeps everything moving smoothly in the blender and determines the overall texture of your drink. The right liquid depends on both your nutritional goals and your flavor preferences.

Here are some options to consider:

- *Water:* If you want a light and refreshing smoothie, plain water is a great option. It's also perfect if you're looking to keep calories low.

- *Almond Milk/Coconut Milk:* For a creamier texture, plant-based milks like almond or coconut milk add richness without dairy. They also bring a subtle nutty or tropical flavor to your smoothie.

- *Greek Yogurt:* If you're looking to add more protein and creaminess, Greek yogurt is a great base. It adds a tangy flavor and a thick consistency, making your smoothie feel more like a meal.

- **_Coconut Water:_** A hydrating, low-calorie option, coconut water is slightly sweet and filled with electrolytes, making it perfect for post-workout smoothies or for days when you need extra hydration.

Tip: Start with about 1 to 1.5 cups of liquid, and you can adjust as needed. If your smoothie ends up too thick, just add a splash more liquid to get the perfect consistency.

2. Pick Your Produce: Fresh or Frozen

One of the best things about smoothies is how easy it is to pack them full of fruits and veggies. And the options are nearly endless. Fresh and frozen produce both work well, so it's all about your preference.

- Frozen fruit is perfect for making thick, icy smoothies. It also eliminates the need for ice, which can sometimes water down your smoothie. Frozen berries, mangoes, or pineapples add sweetness, while bananas create a creamy texture.

- Fresh fruit works best when paired with ice or a frozen ingredient to keep your smoothie chilled. Seasonal fruits like peaches or berries are excellent for adding vibrant flavors.
- Leafy greens like spinach or kale blend seamlessly into smoothies, adding a nutrient boost without altering the flavor too much. If you're new to green smoothies, start with spinach—it's milder in taste compared to kale or other greens.

Tip: A good rule of thumb is to use 1 to 2 cups of fruits and/or veggies per smoothie. And don't be afraid to mix it up—combining fruits with greens makes for a balanced, nutrient-packed smoothie.

3. Add Creaminess with Healthy Fats

The secret to a satisfying smoothie often lies in the creamy texture, which comes from adding healthy fats. These fats not only improve the texture of your smoothie but also keep you fuller for longer and provide essential nutrients.

- *Avocado:* If you've never added avocado to a smoothie, you're in for a treat! It gives a velvety smooth texture without altering the flavor much. Plus, it's packed with heart-healthy fats.
- *Nut Butters:* A tablespoon of peanut butter, almond butter, or cashew butter adds richness, a slight nutty flavor, and protein.
- *Chia Seeds/Flaxseeds:* These tiny seeds are a powerhouse of omega-3 fatty acids and fiber. They thicken your smoothie, making it more satisfying.

Tip: Start with 1/4 to 1/2 an avocado, or a tablespoon of nut butter or seeds, to get that perfect creamy consistency.

4. Don't Forget Protein

Protein is essential, especially if you're using smoothies as a meal replacement or for recovery. It helps build and repair muscles, keeps you full, and adds balance to your smoothie.

- *Greek Yogurt:* Adds both protein and creaminess to your smoothie.
- *Protein Powder:* A scoop of protein powder (whey, plant-based, or collagen) easily boosts the protein content. Just be sure to choose one that fits your dietary needs and flavor preferences.
- *Silken Tofu:* Believe it or not, tofu blends seamlessly into smoothies and is a great plant-based protein option that also adds thickness.

Tip: Aim to add at least 10 to 20 grams of protein to your smoothie, especially if it's replacing a meal.

5. Sweeten (If Needed) the Natural Way

Fruits naturally sweeten smoothies, but if you find you need a little extra sweetness, there are plenty of natural options that won't spike your blood sugar the way refined sugars do.

- *Dates:* These little powerhouses are full of fiber and natural sweetness. Just make sure to pit them before blending!
- *Honey or Maple Syrup:* A teaspoon or two of honey or maple syrup adds a touch of sweetness without overwhelming the flavors.
- *Stevia:* A few drops of liquid stevia can sweeten your smoothie without adding calories or sugar.

Tip: Taste your smoothie before adding extra sweeteners. Sometimes, the fruit itself is all you need!

6. Boost Your Nutrition

Smoothies are the perfect canvas for adding superfoods and nutritional boosts. Here are a few of my favorite options:

- *Spinach or Kale:* Both are loaded with vitamins and blend easily into most smoothies without affecting taste.
- *Chia Seeds/Flaxseeds:* High in fiber and omega-3s, these seeds add a boost of nutrition and help keep you full.
- *Turmeric/Ginger:* Known for their anti-inflammatory properties, these spices can be added for a subtle warmth and healing benefits.
- *Spirulina:* A powerful source of antioxidants and protein, spirulina powder adds a nutrient boost and a vibrant green color to your smoothie.

Tip: Just a teaspoon of any of these boosters is usually all you need for added benefits.

Balancing Flavors and Textures: The Perfect Harmony

Now that you've got all your ingredients, the next step is creating a balance of flavors and textures. This is where smoothie-making becomes an art. Finding the right blend of sweet, creamy, tangy, and refreshing takes some experimentation, but here's how to master it:

1. Balancing Sweetness and Tang

The key to a delicious smoothie is finding the sweet spot (pun intended!) between sweetness and tanginess. Here's how to get it just right:

- *Sweet Fruits:* Bananas, mangoes, and dates bring natural sweetness and smooth texture to your smoothie.
- *Tart Ingredients:* Pineapple, citrus fruits (like oranges and lemons), and Greek yogurt add a tangy twist to cut through sweetness. A splash of lemon

juice can also brighten up flavors and add complexity.

Tip: Start with a sweet base (like banana or mango), then add a splash of tart fruit juice or a squeeze of lemon to balance it out.

2. Mixing Creamy and Icy

Textures are just as important as flavors when it comes to creating a great smoothie. The balance between creamy and icy is what gives your smoothie that satisfying, refreshing texture.

- *Creamy Ingredients:* Avocado, yogurt, nut butters, and frozen bananas are your go-to for creaminess.
- *Icy Ingredients:* Frozen fruits or a handful of ice cubes can create that frosty, refreshing texture.

Tip: For a smoother consistency, skip the ice cubes and rely on frozen fruits instead.

3. Enhance the Flavor with a Dash of Spice

Don't be afraid to spice things up! Spices can take a smoothie from ordinary to extraordinary in just a pinch.

- *Cinnamon:* Adds warmth and depth, especially in smoothies with bananas, apples, or oats.
- *Ginger:* Fresh or powdered ginger adds a refreshing zing and can help with digestion.
- *Vanilla Extract:* Just a drop or two of vanilla can elevate the flavor of your smoothie and make it feel like a dessert.

Tip: A little goes a long way with spices, so start with just a pinch or a few drops.

Ready to Blend the Perfect Smoothie?

Now that you've got the tips and tricks, it's time to create your perfect smoothie. With the right balance of flavors and textures, you can whip up a smoothie that's not only delicious but also packed with nutrients to fuel your body.

Whether you're making a light snack, a post-workout recovery drink, or a full-on meal replacement, smoothies are your blank canvas. Get creative, experiment with flavors, and most importantly—enjoy the process!

Best Smoothie Preparation Techniques

Adapting Recipes for Specific Symptoms

Friendly Guide to Creating Delicious, Healing Smoothies for Pancreatic Cancer

When it comes to preparing smoothies for pancreatic cancer, it's not just about blending fruits and veggies—it's about ensuring every sip helps nourish your body, address specific symptoms, and tastes amazing. Whether you're dealing with nausea, fatigue, or weight loss, we can tweak your smoothie recipes to support your unique needs while keeping them flavorful and easy to enjoy.

Let's dive into some pro tips on how to make the most of your smoothie-making routine!

Best Smoothie Preparation Techniques includes:

1. Choose Your Base Wisely

The liquid base is the foundation of any great smoothie, and you want to choose options that are both nutritious and easy to digest. Here are some go-to choices:

- Coconut water for hydration and electrolytes.
- Almond milk or oat milk for a creamy texture without dairy.
- Herbal teas like ginger or chamomile, which are soothing and gentle on the stomach.

Tip: If you're experiencing bloating or discomfort, stick with lighter bases like coconut water. For those needing extra calories, nut milks are a good option.

2. Focus on Soft, Easy-to-Digest Ingredients

For pancreatic cancer patients, digestion can be sensitive, so using ingredients that are easy to process is key. Opt for soft fruits like bananas, mangoes, or peaches, and use steamed vegetables like carrots or spinach (yes, steamed greens blend much better).

Tip: If you're having trouble with raw ingredients, lightly steaming or boiling them before blending can make them easier to digest without losing nutrients.

3. Incorporate Protein Smoothly

Getting enough protein is important, especially if you're dealing with muscle loss or fatigue. For a smooth consistency, try:

- Nut butters (peanut, almond, cashew) for creaminess and protein.
- Plant-based protein powders like pea or hemp protein, which blend well.
- Silken tofu, which adds a protein boost while staying silky and smooth.

Tip: Avoid gritty protein powders, which can feel heavy or unpleasant. Stick to high-quality, smooth-textured options.

4. Blend in Healthy Fats for Weight Maintenance

Healthy fats can help maintain weight and boost calories without making the smoothie too thick.

Some great fats to blend into your smoothies include:

- Avocado for creaminess and heart-healthy fats.
- Coconut oil or MCT oil, which are easily digestible.

- Ground flaxseeds or chia seeds, which add omega-3s and a slight thickness.

Tip: If you're struggling with weight loss, aim for more calorie-dense ingredients like avocado and coconut milk.

5. Smooth Texture and Temperature Matter

Smoothies should be easy to sip, especially if nausea or throat sensitivity is an issue. Aim for a smooth, lump-free texture. If you prefer a chilled smoothie, use frozen fruits or add ice cubes, but keep it at a moderate chill if cold temperatures are irritating.

Tip: If you're experiencing nausea, smoothies that are closer to room temperature may be easier to tolerate than icy ones.

Adapting Recipes for Specific Symptoms

For Nausea Relief

When nausea hits, the key is to keep your smoothie light, soothing, and not too heavy on the stomach. Try these adjustments:

Ginger is your best friend. Add a small piece of fresh ginger or ginger tea as the base to settle the stomach.

- Stick to mild flavors like bananas and pears, which are less likely to trigger nausea.
- Avoid strong or sour fruits like citrus, which can be too intense.

For Fatigue

When fatigue sets in, energy-boosting ingredients are key. Focus on adding protein and healthy fats to give you sustained energy without causing a crash.

- Nut butters or plant-based protein powder can keep you going.

- Spinach or kale can provide a gentle boost of iron and B vitamins to support energy levels.
- Add some oats or chia seeds for fiber and slow-releasing carbs.

For Weight Loss or Muscle Wasting

If you're struggling with unintentional weight loss, smoothies can be a great way to add extra calories without feeling overwhelmed by large meals.

- Add calorie-dense ingredients like avocados, nut butters, and full-fat coconut milk.
- Protein is important for maintaining muscle mass, so include protein powders or Greek yogurt (if tolerated).
- A touch of honey or maple syrup can sweeten things up while adding extra calories.

Final Tips for Smoothie Success

- *Experiment with small servings first:* If you're unsure how your body will react to certain ingredients, start small and see how you feel.
- *Use fresh, whole ingredients:* Whenever possible, stick with fresh or frozen fruits and veggies to maximize nutrient content.
- *Customize to your taste:* Every person's palate is different—add a little sweetness, or keep it more savory, depending on your preferences!

Remember, smoothies are an easy and fun way to incorporate nutrient-dense foods into your diet, especially when you're dealing with pancreatic cancer. They can be adapted to suit your needs, and with a little creativity, you can enjoy delicious, healing smoothies every day. Try different combinations, listen to your body, and enjoy the process of nourishing yourself in a way that feels good.

Part Three

Energizing Breakfast Smoothie Recipes for Pancreatic Cancer

Smoothies are an excellent breakfast option, especially for those dealing with pancreatic cancer, as they are easy to digest, nutrient-packed, and can be tailored to meet specific nutritional needs. Here are some smoothie recipes that provide energy, boost nutrition, and are gentle on the digestive system.

Creamy Avocado Banana Smoothie

This smoothie provides healthy fats, potassium, and protein, perfect for maintaining energy and muscle strength.

Ingredients:

1/2 ripe avocado

1 banana (preferably frozen)

1 cup almond milk (or any plant-based milk)

1 tablespoon almond butter

1 tablespoon chia seeds

1 teaspoon honey (optional)

Instructions:

Place all ingredients in a blender.

Blend on high until smooth and creamy.

Adjust the consistency with extra almond milk
if needed.

Nutritional Information:

Calories: 330, Protein: 7g, Fat: 19g,
Carbohydrates: 36g, Fiber: 9g

Spinach & Pineapple Power Smoothie

A refreshing blend of spinach and pineapple loaded with vitamins and antioxidants to boost your immune system.

Ingredients:

1 cup fresh spinach

1/2 cup frozen pineapple chunks

1/2 banana

1 cup coconut water

1 tablespoon ground flaxseeds

1 tablespoon fresh lemon juice

Instructions:

Combine spinach, pineapple, banana, coconut water, flaxseeds, and lemon juice in the blender.

Blend until smooth, adding more coconut water for a thinner consistency.

Nutritional Information:

Calories: 180, Protein: 3g, Fat: 4g, Carbohydrates: 38g, Fiber: 7g

Berry Oat Smoothie

This smoothie provides long-lasting energy with a healthy balance of fiber, antioxidants, and protein.

Ingredients:

1/2 cup rolled oats

1/2 cup mixed frozen berries (blueberries, strawberries, raspberries)

1/2 cup Greek yogurt (dairy-free if needed)

1 tablespoon chia seeds

1 cup almond milk

1 teaspoon maple syrup (optional)

Instructions:

Add oats, berries, yogurt, chia seeds, almond milk, and maple syrup to the blender.

Blend until smooth and creamy.

Let it sit for a few minutes to allow the oats to soften.

Nutritional Information:

Calories: 270, Protein: 10g, Fat: 6g, Carbohydrates: 45g, Fiber: 8g

Peanut Butter & Banana Protein Smoothie

Packed with protein and healthy fats, this smoothie is ideal for energy and weight maintenance.

Ingredients:

1 banana

1 tablespoon peanut butter

1 cup unsweetened almond milk

1 tablespoon ground flaxseeds

1 scoop plant-based protein powder (optional)

1/2 teaspoon cinnamon

Instructions:

Blend banana, peanut butter, almond milk, flaxseeds, protein powder, and cinnamon until smooth.

Adjust consistency with more almond milk if needed.

Nutritional Information:

Calories: 350, Protein: 12g, Fat: 14g, Carbohydrates: 45g, Fiber: 8g

Mango Coconut Energy Smoothie

A tropical treat that offers hydration, vitamins, and energy-boosting healthy fats.

Ingredients:

1/2 cup frozen mango chunks

1/2 banana

1 cup coconut milk

1 tablespoon coconut oil

1 teaspoon honey (optional)

Instructions:

Blend mango, banana, coconut milk, coconut oil, and honey until creamy.

Serve immediately and enjoy the tropical flavors.

Nutritional Information:

Calories: 320, Protein: 3g, Fat: 23g, Carbohydrates: 30g, Fiber: 4g

Blueberry Almond Smoothie

This smoothie is rich in antioxidants, healthy fats, and protein, helping to fight fatigue and improve overall well-being.

Ingredients:

1/2 cup frozen blueberries

1/2 banana

1 tablespoon almond butter

1/2 cup almond milk

1 tablespoon ground flaxseeds

Instructions:

Blend blueberries, banana, almond butter, almond milk, and flaxseeds until smooth.

Add more almond milk for a thinner consistency, if needed.

Nutritional Information:

Calories: 280, Protein: 6g, Fat: 14g, Carbohydrates: 36g, Fiber: 8g

Tropical Green Smoothie

This nutrient-dense smoothie helps support digestion and provides essential vitamins.

Ingredients:

1/2 cup fresh spinach

1/2 cup frozen pineapple

1/2 frozen banana

1/2 avocado

1 cup coconut water

1 teaspoon honey (optional)

Instructions:

Blend spinach, pineapple, banana, avocado, and coconut water until smooth.

Add honey to taste and serve chilled.

Nutritional Information:

Calories: 240, Protein: 3g, Fat: 12g, Carbohydrates: 32g, Fiber: 8g

Pumpkin Spice Smoothie

Rich in fiber and vitamins, this smoothie is perfect for a cozy, fall-inspired breakfast.

Ingredients:

1/2 cup canned pumpkin puree

1/2 frozen banana

1 cup unsweetened almond milk

1 tablespoon chia seeds

1/2 teaspoon cinnamon

1/4 teaspoon nutmeg

Instructions:

Blend pumpkin, banana, almond milk, chia seeds, cinnamon, and nutmeg until smooth.

Serve with a dash of cinnamon on top for extra flavor.

Nutritional Information:

Calories: 190, Protein: 4g, Fat: 5g, Carbohydrates: 36g, Fiber: 8g

Apple Cinnamon Oat Smoothie

This smoothie offers a warm, comforting flavor packed with fiber, healthy carbs, and energy.

Ingredients:

1/2 apple (chopped)

1/4 cup rolled oats

1/2 frozen banana

1/2 cup unsweetened almond milk

1 tablespoon almond butter

1/2 teaspoon cinnamon

Instructions:

Blend apple, oats, banana, almond milk, almond butter, and cinnamon until smooth.

Let it sit for a few minutes to soften the oats, then blend again before serving.

Nutritional Information:

Calories: 260, Protein: 6g, Fat: 9g, Carbohydrates: 42g, Fiber: 7g

Carrot & Ginger Smoothie

A vitamin-packed smoothie that helps with digestion and inflammation, perfect for a fresh start to the day.

Ingredients:

1/2 cup steamed carrots

1/2 frozen banana

1/2 teaspoon fresh grated ginger

1 cup orange juice (freshly squeezed)

1 tablespoon chia seeds

Instructions:

Blend carrots, banana, ginger, orange juice, and chia seeds until smooth.

Add more orange juice if a thinner consistency is preferred.

Nutritional Information:

Calories: 210, Protein: 4g, Fat: 5g, Carbohydrates: 42g, Fiber: 7g

These energizing breakfast smoothies are designed to support overall health while helping manage symptoms related to pancreatic cancer. Each recipe is packed with nutrients to keep you feeling energized, nourished, and satisfied throughout the day!

Protein-Packed Smoothies for Muscle Recovery

For Pancreatic Cancer Patients Looking to Support Muscle Health

Protein is crucial for muscle recovery, especially for individuals facing muscle loss or fatigue during pancreatic cancer treatment. These smoothies are designed to provide a rich source of plant-based or gentle proteins, helping to repair and maintain muscle mass while offering easy-to-digest nourishment.

Peanut Butter Banana Protein Smoothie

This smoothie is loaded with plant-based protein and healthy fats to help support muscle recovery and maintain energy levels.

Ingredients:

1 banana (frozen)

1 tablespoon peanut butter (or almond butter)

1 scoop plant-based protein powder (vanilla or unflavored)

1 cup unsweetened almond milk

1 tablespoon chia seeds

1/2 teaspoon vanilla extract

Instructions:

Add all ingredients to the blender.

Blend on high until smooth and creamy.

Adjust thickness by adding more almond milk if needed.

Nutritional Information:

Calories: 390, Protein: 22g, Fat: 18g, Carbohydrates: 38g, Fiber: 9g

Blueberry Almond Protein Smoothie

Blueberries and almond butter offer antioxidants and protein, perfect for muscle recovery and overall wellness.

Ingredients:

1/2 cup frozen blueberries

1 tablespoon almond butter

1/2 cup Greek yogurt (or dairy-free yogurt)

1 scoop plant-based protein powder

1 cup unsweetened almond milk

1 tablespoon ground flaxseeds

Instructions:

Combine all ingredients in the blender.

Blend until smooth and creamy.

Serve immediately and enjoy the refreshing blueberry flavor.

Nutritional Information:

Calories: 350, Protein: 28g, Fat: 15g, Carbohydrates: 27g, Fiber: 7g

Chocolate Avocado Protein Smoothie

Avocado adds creaminess and healthy fats, while chocolate protein powder provides a satisfying flavor and muscle-supporting protein.

Ingredients:

1/2 ripe avocado

1 scoop chocolate protein powder

1 tablespoon unsweetened cocoa powder

1 cup unsweetened almond milk

1 tablespoon chia seeds

1 teaspoon honey (optional)

Instructions:

Add avocado, protein powder, cocoa powder, almond milk, chia seeds, and honey to the blender.

Blend until smooth and creamy.

If desired, add ice cubes for a chilled smoothie.

Nutritional Information:

Calories: 380, Protein: 22g, Fat: 21g, Carbohydrates: 24g, Fiber: 10g

Mango Coconut Protein Smoothie

A tropical smoothie rich in plant-based protein and healthy fats, designed to support muscle recovery and energy levels.

Ingredients:

1/2 cup frozen mango chunks

1/2 banana

1 scoop plant-based protein powder (vanilla)

1 cup coconut milk (full-fat or light)

1 tablespoon coconut oil

1 teaspoon chia seeds

Instructions:

Blend mango, banana, protein powder, coconut milk, coconut oil, and chia seeds until smooth.

Serve immediately for a delicious tropical treat.

Nutritional Information:

Calories: 420, Protein: 20g, Fat: 25g, Carbohydrates: 34g, Fiber: 7g

Pumpkin Spice Protein Smoothie

This seasonal smoothie offers a balance of protein and fiber to help with muscle recovery and digestion.

Ingredients:

1/2 cup canned pumpkin puree

1/2 frozen banana

1 scoop vanilla protein powder

1 cup unsweetened almond milk

1 tablespoon chia seeds

1/2 teaspoon cinnamon

1/4 teaspoon nutmeg

Instructions:

Add pumpkin, banana, protein powder, almond milk, chia seeds, cinnamon, and nutmeg to the blender.

Blend until smooth and creamy.

Enjoy with a dash of extra cinnamon on top for added flavor.

Nutritional Information:

Calories: 320, Protein: 22g, Fat: 8g, Carbohydrates: 44g, Fiber: 10g

Each of these smoothies is specifically designed for individuals undergoing treatment for pancreatic cancer who need to support muscle recovery and maintain energy levels. They are packed with protein, fiber, healthy fats, and essential nutrients, all in a format that is easy to digest and delicious to drink.

Enjoy these protein-packed smoothies as a convenient way to nourish your body and help your muscles heal and rebuild!

Immune-Boosting Smoothie Recipes

For Pancreatic Cancer Patients Seeking Nourishment and Immune Support

Pancreatic cancer treatments can weaken the immune system, making it vital to incorporate foods rich in vitamins, minerals, and antioxidants. These smoothies are designed to boost the immune system while providing essential nutrients in an easy-to-digest format.

Citrus & Ginger Immunity Smoothie

Packed with vitamin C from citrus fruits and anti-inflammatory properties from ginger, this smoothie strengthens the immune system and soothes digestive discomfort.

Ingredients:

1 orange, peeled

1/2 lemon, juiced

1/2 frozen banana

1 teaspoon freshly grated ginger

1 tablespoon chia seeds

1 cup coconut water

Instructions:

Add orange, lemon juice, banana, ginger, chia seeds, and coconut water to the blender.

Blend on high until smooth.

Serve immediately for a refreshing, immune-boosting smoothie.

Nutritional Information:

Calories: 160, Protein: 3g, Fat: 3g, Carbohydrates: 36g, Fiber: 8g

Spinach & Pineapple Green Smoothie

This smoothie combines spinach (rich in vitamins A and C) with pineapple's anti-inflammatory bromelain to promote immune function and overall health.

Ingredients:

1 cup fresh spinach

1/2 cup frozen pineapple chunks

1/2 banana

1 cup unsweetened almond milk

1 tablespoon ground flaxseeds

Instructions:

Add spinach, pineapple, banana, almond milk, and flaxseeds to the blender.

Blend until smooth and creamy.

Adjust thickness by adding more almond milk, if necessary.

Nutritional Information:

Calories: 190, Protein: 4g, Fat: 5g,

Carbohydrates: 35g, Fiber: 6g

Turmeric & Mango Immune Booster

Turmeric, known for its powerful anti-inflammatory and antioxidant properties, pairs with mango's vitamin C to support immune health.

Ingredients:

1/2 cup frozen mango chunks

1/2 banana

1 teaspoon turmeric powder

1/4 teaspoon black pepper (to enhance turmeric absorption)

1/2 cup unsweetened almond milk

1/2 cup coconut water

Instructions:

Combine mango, banana, turmeric, black pepper, almond milk, and coconut water in the blender.

Blend until smooth.

Serve immediately and enjoy the vibrant flavors.

Nutritional Information:

Calories: 180, Protein: 3g, Fat: 3g,

Carbohydrates: 36g, Fiber: 5g

Berry & Beet Immunity Smoothie

Beets and berries are loaded with antioxidants and vitamins, particularly vitamin C, to help boost your immune defenses and fight oxidative stress.

Ingredients:

1/2 cup mixed frozen berries (blueberries, strawberries, raspberries)

1/2 small cooked beet (peeled)

1 tablespoon chia seeds

1/2 cup Greek yogurt (or dairy-free alternative)

1 cup unsweetened almond milk

Instructions:

Add berries, beet, chia seeds, yogurt, and almond milk to the blender.

Blend until smooth and creamy.

Adjust with more almond milk for a thinner consistency.

Nutritional Information:

Calories: 220, Protein: 9g, Fat: 5g, Carbohydrates: 36g, Fiber: 9g

Carrot & Apple Immunity Smoothie

Carrots provide beta-carotene (vitamin A) and apples offer vitamin C, both essential for immune health. This smoothie also contains ginger for its anti-inflammatory benefits.

Ingredients:

1/2 cup chopped carrots (steamed or raw)

1 apple, cored and chopped

1/2 banana

1/2 teaspoon freshly grated ginger

1 cup orange juice (freshly squeezed if possible)

Instructions:

Add carrots, apple, banana, ginger, and orange juice to the blender.

Blend on high until smooth.

Serve chilled for a nutrient-dense, immune-boosting drink.

Nutritional Information:

Calories: 210, Protein: 3g, Fat: 1g, Carbohydrates: 50g, Fiber: 8g

These immune-boosting smoothies are packed with vitamins, antioxidants, and anti-inflammatory ingredients that help support a weakened immune system during pancreatic cancer treatment. Easy to digest and filled with flavor, they can help strengthen your body's defenses while nourishing you from the inside out.

Anti-inflammatory Smoothies for Pain Relief

For Pancreatic Cancer Patients Seeking Natural Pain Management

Chronic inflammation is a common issue during pancreatic cancer treatment, contributing to pain and discomfort. These anti-inflammatory smoothies are packed with ingredients like turmeric, ginger, and berries, known for their pain-relieving and anti-inflammatory properties.

Turmeric & Pineapple Pain Relief Smoothie

Turmeric is a powerful anti-inflammatory spice, while pineapple contains bromelain, an enzyme known to reduce inflammation and pain.

Ingredients:

1/2 cup frozen pineapple chunks

1/2 banana

1 teaspoon turmeric powder

1/2 teaspoon freshly grated ginger

1/4 teaspoon black pepper (to enhance turmeric absorption)

1 cup coconut water

Instructions:

Add pineapple, banana, turmeric, ginger, black pepper, and coconut water to the blender.

Blend on high until smooth.

Serve chilled and enjoy the tropical flavors.

Nutritional Information:

Calories: 160, Protein: 1g, Fat: 1g, Carbohydrates: 38g, Fiber: 5g

Cherry & Ginger Anti-Inflammatory Smoothie

Cherries are rich in anthocyanins, compounds that reduce inflammation, while ginger has long been used for its pain-relieving benefits.

Ingredients:

1/2 cup frozen cherries

1/2 frozen banana

1 teaspoon freshly grated ginger

1 tablespoon chia seeds

1 cup unsweetened almond milk

1/2 teaspoon cinnamon

Instructions:

Combine cherries, banana, ginger, chia seeds, almond milk, and cinnamon in the blender.

Blend until smooth.

Serve immediately and feel the pain-relieving effects of cherries and ginger.

Nutritional Information:

Calories: 180, Protein: 4g, Fat: 4g, Carbohydrates: 34g, Fiber: 7g

Spinach & Blueberry Anti-Inflammatory Smoothie

Blueberries are rich in antioxidants, while spinach offers a wealth of anti-inflammatory nutrients, including vitamin E and polyphenols.

Ingredients:

1 cup fresh spinach

1/2 cup frozen blueberries

1/2 banana

1 tablespoon ground flaxseeds

1 cup unsweetened almond milk

Instructions:

Add spinach, blueberries, banana, flaxseeds, and almond milk to the blender.

Blend until smooth and creamy.

Serve chilled for a nutrient-packed smoothie that fights inflammation.

Nutritional Information:

Calories: 180, Protein: 5g, Fat: 5g, Carbohydrates: 33g, Fiber: 7g

Carrot, Apple & Ginger Inflammation Buster

Carrots provide beta-carotene, a powerful antioxidant, while ginger and apple offer anti-inflammatory benefits to help ease pain.

Ingredients:

1/2 cup chopped carrots (steamed or raw)

1 apple, cored and chopped

1/2 frozen banana

1 teaspoon freshly grated ginger

1 cup unsweetened almond milk

Instructions:

Add carrots, apple, banana, ginger, and almond milk to the blender.

Blend on high until smooth.

Adjust consistency by adding more almond milk if necessary.

Nutritional Information:

Calories: 190, Protein: 3g, Fat: 3g, Carbohydrates: 45g, Fiber: 7g

Beet & Pomegranate Anti-Inflammatory Smoothie

Beets are a fantastic anti-inflammatory food rich in nitrates, and pomegranate provides antioxidants that help reduce inflammation and pain.

Ingredients:

1/2 small cooked beet (peeled)

1/2 cup pomegranate juice

1/2 frozen banana

1 tablespoon chia seeds

1 cup unsweetened almond milk

Instructions:

Add beet, pomegranate juice, banana, chia seeds, and almond milk to the blender.

Blend until smooth and creamy.

Serve immediately for a refreshing smoothie that fights inflammation.

Nutritional Information:

Calories: 200, Protein: 4g, Fat: 5g, Carbohydrates: 38g, Fiber: 6g

These anti-inflammatory smoothies are designed to help ease pain and reduce inflammation during pancreatic cancer treatment. They are rich in natural anti-inflammatory compounds like turmeric, ginger, cherries, and beets, making them an excellent addition to your daily routine to manage discomfort and promote healing.

Smoothies for Nausea and Digestive Comfort

For Pancreatic Cancer Patients Seeking Relief from Nausea and Digestive Issues

Nausea and digestive discomfort are common challenges during pancreatic cancer treatment. These smoothies are gentle on the stomach, providing soothing and easy-to-digest ingredients that help alleviate nausea while still offering essential nutrients.

Ginger & Banana Nausea Relief Smoothie

Ginger is a well-known remedy for nausea, and bananas are easy to digest and gentle on the stomach, making this smoothie perfect for calming digestive discomfort.

Ingredients:

1 frozen banana

1 teaspoon freshly grated ginger

1/2 cup plain Greek yogurt (or dairy-free alternative)

1 tablespoon honey (optional)

1 cup unsweetened almond milk

Instructions:

Add banana, ginger, yogurt, honey, and almond milk to the blender.

Blend on high until smooth and creamy.

Serve chilled for a refreshing and soothing smoothie.

Nutritional Information:

Calories: 230, Protein: 10g, Fat: 4g, Carbohydrates: 44g, Fiber: 4g

Peppermint & Cucumber Digestive Soother

Peppermint is known for its calming effect on the digestive system, and cucumber offers hydration and a light, refreshing flavor to soothe the stomach.

Ingredients:

1/2 cucumber (peeled and chopped)

1/2 frozen banana

1/2 cup coconut water

1 teaspoon peppermint extract (or a few fresh mint leaves)

1/2 cup ice cubes

Instructions:

Add cucumber, banana, coconut water, peppermint extract, and ice cubes to the blender.

Blend until smooth and chilled.

Enjoy this light and refreshing smoothie for digestive comfort.

Nutritional Information:

Calories: 120, Protein: 1g, Fat: 1g, Carbohydrates: 30g, Fiber: 3g

Papaya & Pineapple Digestive Enzyme Smoothie

Papaya and pineapple contain natural enzymes (papain and bromelain) that aid digestion, making this smoothie ideal for easing digestive discomfort and promoting gut health.

Ingredients:

1/2 cup papaya chunks

1/2 cup frozen pineapple chunks

1/2 banana

1 cup coconut water

1 tablespoon chia seeds

Instructions:

Combine papaya, pineapple, banana, coconut water, and chia seeds in the blender.

Blend until smooth and creamy.

Serve immediately for a tropical smoothie that aids digestion.

Nutritional Information:

Calories: 180, Protein: 3g, Fat: 4g, Carbohydrates: 39g, Fiber: 7g

Apple & Ginger Digestive Aid Smoothie

Apples provide gentle fiber and pectin to help soothe the stomach, while ginger helps alleviate nausea, making this smoothie a perfect blend for digestive relief.

Ingredients:

1 apple (cored and chopped)

1 teaspoon freshly grated ginger

1/2 frozen banana

1 cup unsweetened almond milk

1 tablespoon honey (optional)

Instructions:

Add apple, ginger, banana, almond milk, and honey to the blender.

Blend until smooth and creamy.

Serve chilled for a delicious, stomach-calming drink.

Nutritional Information:

Calories: 200, Protein: 2g, Fat: 3g, Carbohydrates: 46g, Fiber: 6g

Melon & Mint Cooling Smoothie

Melons are hydrating and easy to digest, while mint offers a cooling sensation that can help alleviate nausea and settle the stomach.

Ingredients:

1 cup cantaloupe or honeydew melon (chopped)

1/2 frozen banana

1/2 cup coconut water

1 teaspoon fresh mint leaves

1/2 cup ice cubes

Instructions:

Add melon, banana, coconut water, mint leaves, and ice cubes to the blender.

Blend until smooth and creamy.

Serve immediately for a cool and refreshing digestive aid.

Nutritional Information:

Calories: 140, Protein: 2g, Fat: 1g, Carbohydrates: 35g, Fiber: 3g

These smoothies for nausea and digestive comfort are crafted with gentle ingredients like ginger, mint, and easily digestible fruits. They are perfect for individuals experiencing nausea and digestive discomfort during pancreatic cancer treatment, offering a soothing, nutrient-packed option for maintaining nutrition while calming the stomach.

Hydrating Smoothies for Dry Mouth

For Pancreatic Cancer Patients Seeking Relief from Dry Mouth

Dry mouth is a common side effect during pancreatic cancer treatment. These hydrating smoothies are packed with water-rich ingredients like cucumbers, melons, and coconut water to help combat dryness and provide essential hydration, while being gentle on the digestive system.

Cucumber & Aloe Vera Hydration Smoothie

Cucumbers are high in water content, and aloe vera is soothing and hydrating, making this smoothie perfect for dry mouth relief.

Ingredients:

1/2 cucumber (peeled and chopped)

1/4 cup aloe vera juice (make sure it's food-grade)

1/2 frozen banana

1/2 cup coconut water

1 tablespoon honey (optional)

Instructions:

Add cucumber, aloe vera juice, banana, coconut water, and honey to the blender.

Blend on high until smooth and creamy.

Serve chilled for a refreshing, hydrating experience.

Nutritional Information:

Calories: 130, Protein: 1g, Fat: 1g, Carbohydrates: 33g, Fiber: 2g

Watermelon & Mint Cooling Smoothie

Watermelon is incredibly hydrating, with over 90% water content, and mint adds a cooling effect to this smoothie, helping soothe a dry mouth.

Ingredients:

1 cup watermelon cubes (seedless)

1/2 frozen banana

1/2 cup coconut water

1 teaspoon fresh mint leaves

1/2 cup ice cubes

Instructions:

Add watermelon, banana, coconut water, mint leaves, and ice cubes to the blender.

Blend until smooth and refreshing.

Serve immediately to enjoy the cooling and hydrating effects.

Nutritional Information:

Calories: 110, Protein: 1g, Fat: 0g, Carbohydrates: 28g, Fiber: 2g

Cantaloupe & Coconut Water Hydration Smoothie

Cantaloupe is another water-rich fruit, and when paired with coconut water, this smoothie becomes a hydration powerhouse.

Ingredients:

1 cup cantaloupe (chopped)

1/2 cup coconut water

1/2 frozen banana

1 tablespoon chia seeds (optional for extra nutrients)

1/2 cup ice cubes

Instructions:

Add cantaloupe, coconut water, banana, chia seeds, and ice cubes to the blender.

Blend until smooth and creamy.

Serve chilled for a refreshing boost of hydration.

Nutritional Information:

Calories: 150, Protein: 3g, Fat: 3g, Carbohydrates: 32g, Fiber: 6g

Strawberry & Cucumber Hydration Smoothie

Strawberries provide vitamin C and hydration, while cucumber adds an extra boost of water to this refreshing smoothie.

Ingredients:

1/2 cup frozen strawberries

1/2 cucumber (peeled and chopped)

1/2 cup coconut water

1 tablespoon honey (optional)

1/2 cup ice cubes

Instructions:

Add strawberries, cucumber, coconut water, honey, and ice cubes to the blender.

Blend on high until smooth.

Serve immediately for a hydrating and nutrient-rich drink.

Nutritional Information:

Calories: 120, Protein: 1g, Fat: 0g, Carbohydrates: 29g, Fiber: 3g

Honeydew & Lemon Hydrating Smoothie

Honeydew melon is rich in water and electrolytes, and the lemon adds a zesty, refreshing touch that helps stimulate saliva production, making it perfect for relieving dry mouth.

Ingredients:

1 cup honeydew melon (chopped)

1/2 frozen banana

1/2 cup coconut water

1 teaspoon fresh lemon juice

1/2 cup ice cubes

Instructions:

Add honeydew melon, banana, coconut water, lemon juice, and ice cubes to the blender.

Blend until smooth and creamy.

Serve immediately for a hydrating and tangy smoothie.

Nutritional Information:

Calories: 130, Protein: 1g, Fat: 0g, Carbohydrates: 32g, Fiber: 2g

These hydrating smoothies are specially designed to help combat dry mouth by using water-rich ingredients like cucumbers, melons, and coconut water. They are refreshing, easy to digest, and provide essential hydration, while also offering light and natural flavors to help soothe and hydrate the mouth.

High-Calorie Smoothies for Weight Maintenance

For Pancreatic Cancer Patients Needing to Sustain Healthy Weight

Maintaining weight during pancreatic cancer treatment can be challenging, especially with a reduced appetite. These high-calorie smoothies are nutrient-dense, easy to consume, and packed with healthy fats, proteins, and carbohydrates to help maintain or increase weight without putting strain on the digestive system.

Avocado & Peanut Butter Power Smoothie

Avocados and peanut butter are rich in healthy fats and calories, making this smoothie a great option for adding extra energy to your diet.

Ingredients:

1/2 ripe avocado

2 tablespoons peanut butter

1 frozen banana

1 cup whole milk (or dairy-free alternative)

1 tablespoon honey

Instructions:

Add avocado, peanut butter, banana, milk, and honey to the blender.

Blend on high until smooth and creamy.

Serve immediately for a delicious and calorie-packed smoothie.

Nutritional Information:

Calories: 480, Protein: 12g, Fat: 32g, Carbohydrates: 38g, Fiber: 7g

Banana & Oatmeal Breakfast Smoothie

This smoothie combines oats and bananas to provide a carbohydrate boost, while Greek yogurt adds protein and healthy fats.

Ingredients:

1/2 cup rolled oats (soaked in water or milk for 10 minutes)

1 frozen banana

1/2 cup full-fat Greek yogurt

1 cup whole milk

1 tablespoon almond butter

1 teaspoon vanilla extract

Instructions:

Combine soaked oats, banana, yogurt, milk, almond butter, and vanilla extract in the blender.

Blend until smooth.

Enjoy this calorie-rich smoothie for breakfast or a snack.

Nutritional Information:

Calories: 530, Protein: 18g, Fat: 22g, Carbohydrates: 62g, Fiber: 7g

Chocolate Almond Butter Smoothie

This smoothie is perfect for those who want a dessert-like treat while getting a high dose of calories and nutrients.

Ingredients:

2 tablespoons almond butter

1 tablespoon cocoa powder

1 frozen banana

1 cup almond milk (or whole milk)

1 tablespoon honey or maple syrup

Instructions:

Add almond butter, cocoa powder, banana, almond milk, and honey to the blender.

Blend until smooth and creamy.

Serve as a sweet and indulgent high-calorie smoothie.

Nutritional Information:

Calories: 460, Protein: 10g, Fat: 28g, Carbohydrates: 45g, Fiber: 6g

Coconut & Mango Tropical Smoothie

This tropical smoothie brings in calorie-dense ingredients like coconut milk and mango, offering both sweetness and high caloric content.

Ingredients:

1/2 cup coconut milk (full-fat)

1/2 cup frozen mango chunks

1/2 frozen banana

1 tablespoon chia seeds

1 tablespoon honey

Instructions:

Add coconut milk, mango, banana, chia seeds, and honey to the blender.

Blend until smooth and thick.

Enjoy the tropical flavors while boosting your calorie intake.

Nutritional Information:

Calories: 450, Protein: 5g, Fat: 32g, Carbohydrates: 42g, Fiber: 5g

Berry & Nut Protein Smoothie

A combination of mixed berries, nuts, and protein powder makes this smoothie not only high in calories but also rich in antioxidants and muscle-supporting protein.

Ingredients:

1/2 cup mixed frozen berries

1 tablespoon almond butter

1 scoop protein powder (vanilla or unflavored)

1 cup whole milk

1 tablespoon honey or agave syrup

1 tablespoon ground flaxseeds (optional)

Instructions:

Add mixed berries, almond butter, protein powder, milk, honey, and flaxseeds to the blender.

Blend until smooth and creamy.

Serve chilled for a nutritious and calorie-dense smoothie.

Nutritional Information:

Calories: 510, Protein: 25g, Fat: 22g, Carbohydrates: 48g, Fiber: 9g

These high-calorie smoothies are ideal for maintaining or gaining weight during pancreatic cancer treatment. They offer a balanced mix of healthy fats, proteins, and carbohydrates while being easy on digestion. Perfect for individuals who need calorie-dense meals in a convenient and drinkable form.

Smoothies Rich In Healthy Fats

Here are some smoothies rich in healthy fats, specifically designed for supporting pancreatic health and providing essential nutrients:

Creamy Avocado & Spinach Smoothie

This smoothie is packed with heart-healthy fats from avocado and flaxseed oil, while the spinach provides essential vitamins and minerals, especially iron. The chia seeds also add fiber and omega-3s, making it a powerhouse smoothie for those in recovery.

Ingredients:

1/2 ripe avocado

1 cup fresh spinach

1 cup unsweetened almond milk (or any plant-based milk)

1 tablespoon chia seeds

1 tablespoon flaxseed oil (or flaxseeds)

1/2 banana (for natural sweetness)

1/2 teaspoon vanilla extract (optional)

Instructions:

Combine the almond milk, avocado, spinach, chia seeds, flaxseed oil, and banana in a blender.

Blend until smooth and creamy, about 1-2 minutes.

If the smoothie is too thick, add more almond milk to adjust consistency.

Serve immediately for best freshness.

Nutritional Information:

Calories: 280, Protein: 5g, Fat: 20g, Carbs: 24g

Coconut & Almond Butter Smoothie

This recipe is rich in healthy fats from coconut milk and almond butter, this smoothie is not only filling but also hydrating. Coconut milk is a great source of medium-chain triglycerides (MCTs), which are easier to digest and provide a quick energy source.

Ingredients:

1 cup unsweetened coconut milk

1 tablespoon almond butter

1 tablespoon shredded unsweetened coconut

1/2 frozen banana

1 tablespoon chia seeds

1 teaspoon honey (optional)

Instructions:

Place the coconut milk, almond butter, banana, shredded coconut, and chia seeds in a blender.

Blend until smooth and creamy.

Taste and adjust sweetness by adding honey if desired.

Serve chilled.

Nutritional Information:

Calories: 320, Protein: 6g, Fat: 24g, Carbs: 22g

Banana & Walnut Power Smoothie

This smoothie is packed with brain-boosting omega-3 fatty acids from walnuts and flaxseeds, while Greek yogurt adds a protein punch. It's creamy, slightly nutty, and perfect for a nutritious start to the day.

Ingredients:

1 ripe banana

1 tablespoon walnut butter (or 6-8 raw walnuts)

1/2 cup plain Greek yogurt

1 cup unsweetened almond milk

1 tablespoon flaxseeds

1/4 teaspoon cinnamon

Instructions:

Blend the banana, walnut butter, Greek yogurt, almond milk, flaxseeds, and cinnamon in a blender.

Blend until everything is well combined and smooth.

Add more almond milk for a thinner consistency if desired.

Pour into a glass and enjoy!

Nutritional Information:

Calories: 350, Protein: 12g, Fat: 20g, Carbs: 30g

Berry & Hemp Seed Smoothie

Hemp seeds are a great source of plant-based protein and omega-3 and omega-6 fatty acids. This smoothie is rich in antioxidants from the berries, while the avocado adds creaminess and healthy fats.

Ingredients:

1/2 cup frozen mixed berries (blueberries, strawberries, raspberries)

1 tablespoon hemp seeds

1/2 ripe avocado

1 cup unsweetened almond milk

1/2 cup plain Greek yogurt

1 teaspoon honey (optional)

Instructions:

Add the frozen berries, hemp seeds, avocado, almond milk, Greek yogurt, and honey to a blender.

Blend until smooth and creamy.

Serve immediately for a refreshing, nutrient-packed smoothie.

Nutritional Information:

Calories: 290, Protein: 8g, Fat: 18g, Carbs: 28g

Peanut Butter & Oat Smoothie

This smoothie is perfect for sustained energy. The oats provide complex carbohydrates, while peanut butter offers a dose of protein and healthy fats. Flaxseeds further boost the fiber content and provide essential fatty acids, making this smoothie both filling and nourishing.

Ingredients:

1 tablespoon peanut butter (or almond butter)

1/2 cup oats (soaked in water for 10 minutes)

1 cup unsweetened almond milk

1/2 frozen banana

1 tablespoon flaxseeds

1 teaspoon honey (optional)

Instructions:

Drain the soaked oats and add them to the blender along with peanut butter, almond milk, frozen banana, flaxseeds, and honey.

Blend until the mixture is smooth and well combined.

Adjust consistency with more almond milk if needed and serve immediately.

Nutritional Information:

Calories: 350, Protein: 10g, Fat: 15g, Carbs: 40g

These smoothie recipes are designed to provide essential nutrients, healthy fats, and energy while being gentle on the digestive system—ideal for those recovering from pancreatic cancer or looking to support their overall health.

Gentle Detox Smoothie Recipes

Here are some gentle detox smoothie recipes designed to support liver health while being mindful of pancreatic cancer recovery. These smoothies are nutrient-dense, easy on the digestive system, and contain liver-supporting ingredients like leafy greens, citrus fruits, and antioxidant-rich vegetables.

Citrus & Ginger Detox Smoothie

Grapefruit and lemon are high in vitamin C and known for their detoxifying effects on the liver. Ginger helps soothe the digestive system, while chia seeds provide a small amount of healthy fats and fiber to aid in digestion and detoxification.

Ingredients:

1/2 grapefruit, peeled and segmented

1/2 lemon, juiced

1 small cucumber, chopped

1/2-inch piece of fresh ginger, peeled

1 tablespoon chia seeds

1/2 cup coconut water

1/2 cup ice cubes

Instructions:

Add all ingredients—grapefruit, lemon juice, cucumber, ginger, chia seeds, coconut water, and ice—into a blender.

Blend on high until smooth, about 1-2 minutes.

Pour into a glass and serve immediately.

Nutritional Information:

Calories: 110, Protein: 2g, Fat: 4g, Carbs: 22g

Green Apple & Spinach Detox Smoothie

This green smoothie combines the liver-cleansing properties of spinach and celery with the fiber and antioxidants from green apple. Flaxseeds add a dose of healthy fats, which support overall detoxification.

Ingredients:

1 green apple, cored and chopped

1 cup fresh spinach

1/2 celery stalk, chopped

1/2 cucumber, peeled and chopped

1/2 lemon, juiced

1/2 cup unsweetened almond milk

1 tablespoon flaxseeds

Instructions:

Place all ingredients—green apple, spinach, celery, cucumber, lemon juice, almond milk, and flaxseeds—into a blender.

Blend until the mixture is smooth and creamy.

If it's too thick, add more almond milk or water to thin it out.

Serve immediately for a refreshing liver-supporting smoothie.

Nutritional Information:

Calories: 150, Protein: 3g, Fat: 4g, Carbs: 29g

Beet & Carrot Liver Cleanse Smoothie

Beets are known for their ability to support liver detoxification, thanks to betaine, which helps remove toxins from the liver. Carrots provide beta-carotene, while apple adds fiber and sweetness, making this a powerful detox drink.

Ingredients:

1 small beet, peeled and chopped

1 small carrot, peeled and chopped

1/2 apple, cored and chopped

1 tablespoon lemon juice

1/2 cup unsweetened almond milk

1/4 cup ice cubes

Instructions:

Place the chopped beet, carrot, apple, lemon juice, almond milk, and ice cubes into a blender.

Blend until smooth and creamy, about 1-2 minutes.

Serve immediately for a nutrient-rich smoothie.

Nutritional Information:

Calories: 120, Protein: 2g, Fat: 2g, Carbs: 24g

Turmeric & Pineapple Anti-Inflammatory Smoothie

Turmeric is a powerful anti-inflammatory spice that helps the liver detoxify. Paired with pineapple, which contains bromelain (an enzyme that aids digestion), this smoothie is refreshing and supports both liver and pancreatic health.

Ingredients:

1/2 cup fresh or frozen pineapple chunks

1/2 banana

1/2 teaspoon ground turmeric (or a small piece of fresh turmeric)

1/4 teaspoon black pepper (to activate turmeric)

1 tablespoon hemp seeds

1/2 cup coconut water

1/2 cup ice cubes

Instructions:

Add the pineapple, banana, turmeric, black pepper, hemp seeds, coconut water, and ice into a blender.

Blend until smooth and creamy.

Serve immediately for a refreshing anti-inflammatory liver-support smoothie.

Nutritional Information:

Calories: 160, Protein: 4g, Fat: 6g, Carbs: 24g

Avocado & Kale Detox Smoothie

Avocado provides healthy fats that are essential for liver function, while kale is rich in chlorophyll, which helps neutralize toxins. Cucumber and green apple contribute hydration and fiber, making this a perfect detox smoothie for liver and overall health.

Ingredients:

1/2 ripe avocado

1 cup fresh kale leaves (stems removed)

1/2 cucumber, peeled and chopped

1/2 green apple, chopped

1 tablespoon lemon juice

1 cup unsweetened almond milk

1/2 cup ice cubes

Instructions:

Combine all ingredients—avocado, kale, cucumber, green apple, lemon juice, almond milk, and ice—into a blender.

Blend on high until smooth and creamy, about 1-2 minutes.

Pour into a glass and enjoy.

Nutritional Information:

Calories: 210, Protein: 5g, Fat: 14g, Carbs: 20g

These smoothies offer a gentle, natural way to support liver detoxification while ensuring they remain easy to digest and nourishing for those recovering from pancreatic cancer. The recipes are also rich in antioxidants, healthy fats, and essential nutrients to support the body's detox and healing processes.

Low-Sugar, Cleansing Green Smoothie Recipes

Here are some gentle, low-sugar, cleansing green smoothie recipes designed to support pancreatic cancer recovery. These smoothies focus on low-sugar ingredients, greens, and detoxifying elements, while being easy on the digestive system.

Cucumber & Mint Detox Smoothie

This smoothie is hydrating and gentle, with cucumber and coconut water providing electrolytes. The mint and lemon add a refreshing taste while promoting digestion and detoxification.

Ingredients:

1 small cucumber, peeled and chopped

1/2 cup fresh spinach leaves

5 fresh mint leaves

1 tablespoon chia seeds

1/2 lemon, juiced

1/2 cup unsweetened coconut water

1/2 cup ice cubes

Instructions:

Add cucumber, spinach, mint leaves, chia seeds, lemon juice, coconut water, and ice to a blender.

Blend on high until smooth and well combined.

Serve immediately for a refreshing and cleansing drink.

Nutritional Information:

Calories: 50, Protein: 2g, Fat: 2g, Carbs: 9g, Sugar: 3g

Kale & Avocado Creamy Green Smoothie

Avocado adds healthy fats and creaminess to this smoothie, while kale provides detoxifying chlorophyll and antioxidants. This is a nutrient-dense, low-sugar option that helps with digestion and inflammation.

Ingredients:

1/2 ripe avocado

1 cup fresh kale leaves (stems removed)

1/2 cucumber, peeled and chopped

1 tablespoon flaxseeds

1/2 lemon, juiced

1 cup unsweetened almond milk

1/4 cup ice cubes

Instructions:

Place avocado, kale, cucumber, flaxseeds, lemon juice, almond milk, and ice in a blender.

Blend on high until smooth and creamy.

Adjust consistency with more almond milk if needed and serve immediately.

Nutritional Information:

Calories: 180, Protein: 4g, Fat: 14g, Carbs: 11g, Sugar: 1g

Spinach & Ginger Zing Smoothie

This low-sugar smoothie features fresh ginger for an anti-inflammatory kick and spinach for detox support. Green apple adds just enough sweetness without spiking sugar levels, making this a gentle and healing drink.

Ingredients:

1 cup fresh spinach

1 small piece of fresh ginger (about 1/2 inch), peeled

1/2 green apple, cored and chopped

1/2 celery stalk, chopped

1 tablespoon hemp seeds

1/2 cup unsweetened almond milk

1/2 cup water

Instructions:

Add spinach, ginger, green apple, celery, hemp seeds, almond milk, and water to a blender.

Blend until smooth and creamy, about 1-2 minutes.

Serve immediately for the best freshness.

Nutritional Information:

Calories: 110, Protein: 4g, Fat: 5g, Carbs: 14g, Sugar: 5g

Zucchini & Celery Detox Smoothie

Zucchini and celery are light, hydrating vegetables that support digestion and detox. Parsley is rich in antioxidants and helps cleanse the body. This smoothie is low in sugar and packed with fiber.

Ingredients:

1 small zucchini, chopped

1/2 celery stalk, chopped

1/2 cup fresh parsley

1/2 lemon, juiced

1 tablespoon chia seeds

1/2 cup unsweetened coconut water

1/2 cup ice cubes

Instructions:

Combine the zucchini, celery, parsley, lemon juice, chia seeds, coconut water, and ice in a blender.

Blend until smooth and well combined.

Adjust the consistency with more coconut water if needed and serve.

Nutritional Information:

Calories: 70, Protein: 2g, Fat: 3g, Carbs: 10g, Sugar: 2g

Spinach & Cucumber Green Cleanser

This smoothie is hydrating and anti-inflammatory, thanks to turmeric. The spinach provides detoxifying nutrients, while the lime adds a zesty flavor without raising sugar content. It's a perfect, light option for liver and pancreas support.

Ingredients:

1 cup fresh spinach

1 small cucumber, peeled and chopped

1/2 cup unsweetened coconut water

1 tablespoon ground flaxseeds

1/2 lime, juiced

1/4 teaspoon turmeric powder

1/2 cup ice cubes

Instructions:

Place spinach, cucumber, coconut water, flaxseeds, lime juice, turmeric, and ice in a blender.

Blend on high until smooth and creamy.

Serve immediately for a refreshing and anti-inflammatory drink.

Nutritional Information:

Calories: 60, Protein: 2g, Fat: 2g, Carbs: 8g, Sugar: 2g

These low-sugar, cleansing green smoothies are designed to gently detoxify the body while being mindful of sugar intake, making them ideal for pancreatic health. They are loaded with fiber, healthy fats, and essential nutrients to support healing and detoxification.

Vitamin-Packed Smoothie Recipes

Here are some gentle, vitamin-packed smoothie recipes designed to support immune health while being easy on the digestive system. These smoothies are full of essential vitamins, antioxidants, and healing ingredients that are particularly beneficial for those recovering from pancreatic cancer.

Berry & Spinach Immune Booster Smoothie

Berries are packed with antioxidants, particularly vitamin C, which helps boost immune function. Spinach adds a wealth of vitamins like vitamin A and K, while chia seeds provide omega-3 fatty acids and fiber for overall health.

Ingredients:

1/2 cup mixed berries (strawberries, blueberries, raspberries)

1/2 cup fresh spinach leaves

1/2 banana

1/4 cup unsweetened almond milk

1 tablespoon chia seeds

1/2 cup ice cubes

Instructions:

Add berries, spinach, banana, almond milk, chia seeds, and ice to a blender.

Blend on high until smooth and well combined, about 1-2 minutes.

Pour into a glass and enjoy immediately.

Nutritional Information:

Calories: 140, Protein: 3g, Fat: 4g, Carbs: 27g, Sugar: 12g

Orange & Carrot Immune Power Smoothie

Oranges are loaded with vitamin C, while carrots provide beta-carotene, which supports immune function and skin health. Turmeric adds an anti-inflammatory boost, making this smoothie a powerhouse for immunity.

Ingredients:

1 small orange, peeled and segmented

1 small carrot, peeled and chopped

1/2 banana

1/2 cup unsweetened almond milk

1 tablespoon ground flaxseeds

1/4 teaspoon turmeric powder

1/4 cup ice cubes

Instructions:

Add orange, carrot, banana, almond milk, flaxseeds, turmeric, and ice to a blender.

Blend until smooth and creamy.

Serve immediately for a vibrant, immune-boosting smoothie.

Nutritional Information:

Calories: 160, Protein: 3g, Fat: 5g, Carbs: 28g, Sugar: 16g

Kiwi & Kale Vitamin C Smoothie

Kiwi is high in vitamin C and antioxidants, which are crucial for a strong immune system. Kale adds additional vitamins A, C, and K, while hemp seeds provide healthy fats and protein to support immune health and overall body function.

Ingredients:

1 ripe kiwi, peeled and chopped

1/2 cup fresh kale leaves (stems removed)

1/2 green apple, chopped

1/4 cup unsweetened coconut water

1 tablespoon hemp seeds

1/2 cup ice cubes

Instructions:

Place the kiwi, kale, green apple, coconut water, hemp seeds, and ice into a blender.

Blend on high until smooth, about 1-2 minutes.

Serve immediately for a refreshing, immune-boosting drink.

Nutritional Information:

Calories: 130, Protein: 4g, Fat: 4g, Carbs: 23g, Sugar: 13g

Pineapple & Ginger Immune Elixir Smoothie

Pineapple contains bromelain, an enzyme that aids digestion and reduces inflammation, while also being rich in vitamin C. Fresh ginger has powerful anti-inflammatory properties, making this smoothie a perfect choice for immune support and digestive health.

Ingredients:

1/2 cup fresh or frozen pineapple chunks

1/2-inch piece fresh ginger, peeled

1/2 cup fresh spinach leaves

1/2 cup unsweetened coconut water

1 tablespoon ground flaxseeds

1/2 cup ice cubes

Instructions:

Combine the pineapple, ginger, spinach, coconut water, flaxseeds, and ice in a blender.

Blend on high until smooth and well combined.

Serve immediately for a tropical and immune-supportive drink.

Nutritional Information:

Calories: 120, Protein: 2g, Fat: 3g, Carbs: 22g, Sugar: 12g

Mango & Turmeric Anti-Inflammatory Smoothie

Mango is rich in vitamins A and C, essential for immune health. Turmeric adds a strong anti-inflammatory benefit, while chia seeds contribute healthy fats, fiber, and protein, making this smoothie both nourishing and beneficial for overall well-being.

Ingredients:

1/2 cup fresh or frozen mango chunks

1/2 banana

1/2 teaspoon ground turmeric

1 tablespoon chia seeds

1/2 cup unsweetened almond milk

1/2 cup ice cubes

Instructions:

Add the mango, banana, turmeric, chia seeds, almond milk, and ice into a blender.

Blend on high until smooth and creamy.

Pour into a glass and enjoy immediately.

Nutritional Information:

Calories: 160, Protein: 3g, Fat: 4g, Carbs: 29g, Sugar: 18g

These smoothies are loaded with vitamins, particularly vitamin C and antioxidants, that help support and strengthen the immune system. They are low in sugar, easy to digest, and designed to be gentle on the body, making them ideal for pancreatic cancer recovery and general immune health.

Smoothies For Post-Treatment

Here are smoothies specifically designed for post-treatment recovery for individuals with pancreatic cancer. These smoothies focus on gentle, easily digestible ingredients while providing essential nutrients for healing and energy.

Banana & Oatmeal Replenishing Smoothie

This smoothie provides a gentle source of carbohydrates and fiber from the banana and oats, which help restore energy. Almond butter adds healthy fats and protein for post-treatment healing, while cinnamon and vanilla give it a comforting flavor.

Ingredients:

1 small banana, ripe

1/4 cup rolled oats

1/2 cup unsweetened almond milk

1 tablespoon almond butter

1/2 teaspoon cinnamon

1/4 teaspoon vanilla extract

1/2 cup ice cubes

Instructions:

Add the banana, oats, almond milk, almond butter, cinnamon, vanilla, and ice to a blender.

Blend on high until smooth and creamy.

Pour into a glass and enjoy immediately.

Nutritional Information:

Calories: 250, Protein: 5g, Fat: 9g, Carbs: 40g, Sugar: 12g

Avocado & Blueberry Healing Smoothie

Avocado provides healthy fats, which are essential for tissue repair and immune support. Blueberries are rich in antioxidants and vitamins that promote recovery, and flaxseeds offer omega-3 fatty acids to reduce inflammation.

Ingredients:

1/2 ripe avocado

1/2 cup blueberries (fresh or frozen)

1 tablespoon ground flaxseeds

1/2 cup unsweetened coconut water

1/2 cup ice cubes

1/2 teaspoon honey (optional)

Instructions:

Place the avocado, blueberries, flaxseeds, coconut water, ice, and honey into a blender.

Blend on high until smooth and creamy.

Serve immediately for a nutrient-packed recovery drink.

Nutritional Information:

Calories: 210, Protein: 3g, Fat: 12g, Carbs: 25g, Sugar: 10g

Mango & Spinach Energizing Smoothie

Mango is rich in vitamin C and A, aiding in tissue repair and immune support. Spinach adds vital minerals like iron and magnesium for energy, while chia seeds contribute fiber and healthy fats for sustained energy.

Ingredients:

1/2 cup fresh or frozen mango chunks

1 cup fresh spinach leaves

1/2 cup unsweetened almond milk

1 tablespoon chia seeds

1/2 banana

1/4 cup ice cubes

Instructions:

Add the mango, spinach, almond milk, chia seeds, banana, and ice to a blender.

Blend on high until smooth and well combined.

Pour into a glass and enjoy this refreshing, energizing smoothie.

Nutritional Information:

Calories: 170, Protein: 3g, Fat: 6g, Carbs: 30g, Sugar: 17g

Peach & Turmeric Anti-Inflammatory Smoothie

Peaches are soft and gentle on the digestive system, providing vitamins and antioxidants for recovery. Turmeric's anti-inflammatory properties help reduce treatment-related inflammation, while Greek yogurt adds protein for tissue repair.

Ingredients:

1 ripe peach, chopped (or 1/2 cup frozen peaches)

1/2 teaspoon ground turmeric

1 tablespoon hemp seeds

1/2 cup unsweetened almond milk

1/4 cup plain Greek yogurt

1/2 cup ice cubes

Instructions:

Combine peach, turmeric, hemp seeds, almond milk, yogurt, and ice in a blender.

Blend until smooth and creamy, about 1-2 minutes.

Serve immediately for a soothing and nutritious drink.

Nutritional Information:

Calories: 190, Protein: 7g, Fat: 8g, Carbs: 24g, Sugar: 17g

Papaya & Ginger Digestive Smoothie

Papaya contains papain, an enzyme that aids digestion, making it perfect for those recovering from treatments. Ginger helps soothe the stomach, and kefir or yogurt provides probiotics that support gut health, helping the digestive system recover.

Ingredients:

1/2 cup fresh or frozen papaya chunks

1/2-inch piece fresh ginger, peeled

1 tablespoon ground flaxseeds

1/2 cup unsweetened coconut water

1/2 cup plain kefir or Greek yogurt

1/2 cup ice cubes

Instructions:

Add papaya, ginger, flaxseeds, coconut water, kefir, and ice to a blender.

Blend on high until smooth and well combined.

Serve immediately for a smoothie that promotes gentle digestion.

Nutritional Information:

Calories: 170, Protein: 6g, Fat: 5g, Carbs: 25g, Sugar: 15g

These smoothies are designed to be gentle on the digestive system while packing a powerful punch of vitamins, minerals, healthy fats, and proteins essential for recovery. They provide energy, reduce inflammation, and support tissue repair and digestion—key aspects of post-treatment recovery.

Part Three

Rebuilding Strength After Treatment for Pancreatic Cancer

A Comprehensive Guide

Recovering from pancreatic cancer treatment is a journey that requires both patience and strategic planning. Whether it's surgery, chemotherapy, radiation, or a combination of treatments, the body endures immense stress, making the recovery period essential for rebuilding strength, nourishing the body, and regaining energy. Smoothies can play a key role in this recovery by providing easily digestible, nutrient-dense meals that support healing and boost energy levels.

Understanding Post-Treatment Challenges

After pancreatic cancer treatment, the body's nutritional needs shift dramatically. Common side effects such as fatigue, weight loss, nausea, digestive issues, and loss of appetite can make it difficult to eat regular meals.

Additionally, treatments may impact the body's ability to absorb nutrients, particularly fats, proteins, and fat-soluble vitamins, making it crucial to consume nutrient-dense foods that are easy to digest and absorb.

For many recovering patients, eating solid foods can be challenging, and there may be restrictions on what the digestive system can comfortably process. This is where smoothies come in — they offer a convenient and gentle way to nourish the body with minimal digestive strain while delivering essential vitamins, minerals, proteins, and healthy fats.

Key Nutrients to Include in Recovery Smoothies

1. Protein Sources

- **Greek Yogurt:** Provides high-quality protein and probiotics to support digestion and gut health.
- **Protein Powders:** Plant-based or whey protein powders can easily be added to smoothies to increase protein intake, essential for muscle repair and tissue healing.
- **Nuts and Nut Butters:** Almonds, cashews, and peanut butter provide healthy fats and protein that aid in recovery.
- **Tofu or Silken Tofu:** An excellent, mild-tasting addition for boosting protein content in a smoothie.

2. Healthy Fats

- **Avocado:** Adds creaminess to smoothies and is a rich source of monounsaturated fats, which are heart-healthy and anti-inflammatory.
- ***Chia Seeds and Flaxseeds:*** High in omega-3 fatty acids, these seeds help reduce inflammation and support immune function.
- ***Coconut Oil or MCT Oil:*** Quick sources of energy that are easier to digest for those struggling with fat absorption.

3. Fiber & Antioxidants

- ***Berries (Blueberries, Strawberries, Raspberries):*** Rich in antioxidants, which help fight inflammation and repair cellular damage.
- ***Leafy Greens (Spinach, Kale):*** Provide essential vitamins like A, C, and K, and minerals like magnesium for muscle function and recovery.

- ***Oats or Oatmeal:*** Add fiber to smoothies, which helps stabilize blood sugar and provides long-lasting energy.

4. Hydration & Electrolytes

- ***Coconut Water:*** A natural source of electrolytes like potassium, which helps maintain hydration and prevent cramping.
- ***Unsweetened Almond Milk:*** Adds creaminess without excess sugar, making it a gentle liquid base for smoothies.
- ***Cucumber and Watermelon:*** Both are hydrating ingredients that can help replenish fluids lost during treatment.

After pancreatic cancer treatment, rebuilding strength is a gradual process that requires the right nutrition. Smoothies, with their flexibility and nutrient density, are a powerful tool in this recovery journey.

By carefully selecting ingredients that promote healing, energy, and strength, you can fuel your body while giving it the gentle nourishment it needs to heal and thrive post-treatment.

Whether you're focusing on adding protein for muscle repair, fats for brain function and energy, or antioxidants to reduce inflammation, smoothies are a convenient and delicious way to meet your nutritional needs and rebuild your strength after pancreatic cancer treatment.

Conclusion

Embracing Nourishment and Healing with Smoothies for Pancreatic Cancer

The journey of recovery from pancreatic cancer treatment is undoubtedly challenging, but it is also a time of renewal, reflection, and self-care. Nutrition plays a vital role in this process, providing the body with the fuel it needs to heal, regain strength, and thrive.

Throughout this book, we've explored the incredible potential of smoothies as a gentle, yet powerful tool in supporting healing, rebuilding energy, and enhancing overall well-being for those affected by pancreatic cancer.

The Healing Power of Smoothies

Smoothies offer an incredibly versatile and easy way to deliver a wide array of essential nutrients. For individuals recovering from pancreatic cancer treatment, where digestive comfort, nutrient absorption, and energy replenishment are of utmost importance, smoothies provide a convenient solution. With their ability to blend nourishing ingredients into an easily digestible form, smoothies allow the body to receive the nourishment it needs without overwhelming the digestive system.

Each recipe in this book was crafted with care, focusing on ingredients that provide:

- Gentle digestion, making it easier to consume nutrients.
- Anti-inflammatory properties, reducing the impact of treatment on the body.
- Essential vitamins and minerals, supporting immune function, energy production, and cellular repair.
- Proteins and healthy fats, essential for rebuilding muscle mass, tissue recovery, and sustained energy.

By combining fruits, vegetables, protein sources, and healthy fats, these smoothies deliver balanced nutrition that not only aids in physical recovery but also nurtures the mind and soul.

A Personalized Approach to Wellness

One of the key strengths of smoothies is their adaptability. Whether you are looking to boost your energy, improve digestion, or simply enjoy a nutrient-packed snack, smoothies can be tailored to your specific needs. The recipes provided in this book are only a starting point, feel free to experiment with flavors, ingredients, and textures that resonate with your unique preferences and nutritional goals.

For those facing dietary challenges or restrictions, smoothies are also a way to include essential nutrients that might be hard to obtain through solid foods. They can be customized for low-sugar diets, high-protein needs, or even to include immune-boosting ingredients to support recovery and well-being. This flexibility allows for a personalized approach to nutrition that meets your evolving needs throughout the recovery process.

Beyond the Recipes: Building Healthy Habits

While this book is filled with nutritious smoothie recipes, its true purpose is to empower you to take control of your health through mindful, balanced nutrition.

Incorporating smoothies into your daily routine is a simple step toward building sustainable, healthy habits that promote healing and long-term well-being.

Nutrition is not a one-time fix — it is an ongoing journey. As you continue to heal and regain strength, you may find that your nutritional needs evolve. Let these smoothies serve as a foundation for continued nourishment, helping you rebuild strength, support your immune system, and maintain a healthy balance.

Recovery from pancreatic cancer is a deeply personal experience, but you do not have to navigate it alone. By making thoughtful choices about your diet and taking the time to care for your body, you are actively contributing to your healing process.

The recipes and insights in this book are meant to support and guide you, offering a comforting, nutritious, and delicious way to nurture your body as you rebuild your health.

As you blend your next smoothie, take a moment to celebrate the small victories along your journey. Each sip represents a step forward in your recovery — a step toward regaining strength, vitality, and balance. Let these smoothies be a source of nourishment not only for your body but also for your spirit, reminding you of the resilience and healing power that resides within you.

Thank you for allowing this book to be a part of your healing journey. We hope that the recipes, nutritional insights, and tips provided here help you to feel empowered, nourished, and supported throughout your recovery. Remember, healing is a process that takes time, and every step you take toward better nutrition and self-care is a step toward wellness and strength.

Wishing you health, vitality, and peace on your path to recovery.

Made in the USA
Middletown, DE
01 November 2024